Jerry Lee Hutchens

Total Cleansing

Learn the Secrets for Effective Detox

books Alive

Summertown
Tennessee

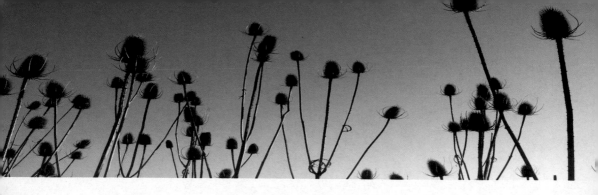

c o n t e n t s

Total Cleansing

Note: Conversions in this book (from imperial to metric) are not exact. They have been rounded to the nearest measurement for convenience. Exact measurements are given in imperial. The recipes in this book are by no means to be taken as therapeutic. They simply promote the philosophy of both the author and *alive* books in relation to whole foods, health and nutrition, while incorporating the practical advice given by the author in the first section of the book.

Recipes

It is your constitutional right to educate yourself in health and medical knowledge, to seek helpful information and make use of it for your own benefit, and for that of your family. You are the one responsible for your health. In order to make decisions in all health matters, you must educate yourself. With this book and the guidance of a naturopath or alternative medical doctor, you will learn what is needed to achieve optimal health.

Those individuals currently taking pharmaceutical prescription drugs will want to talk to their health care professional about the negative effects that the drugs can have on herbal remedies and nutritional supplements, before combining them.

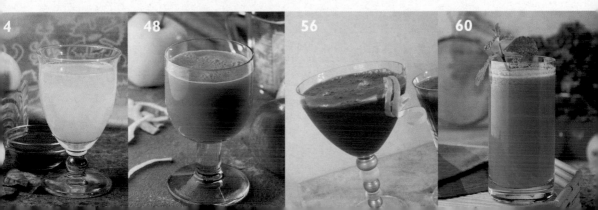

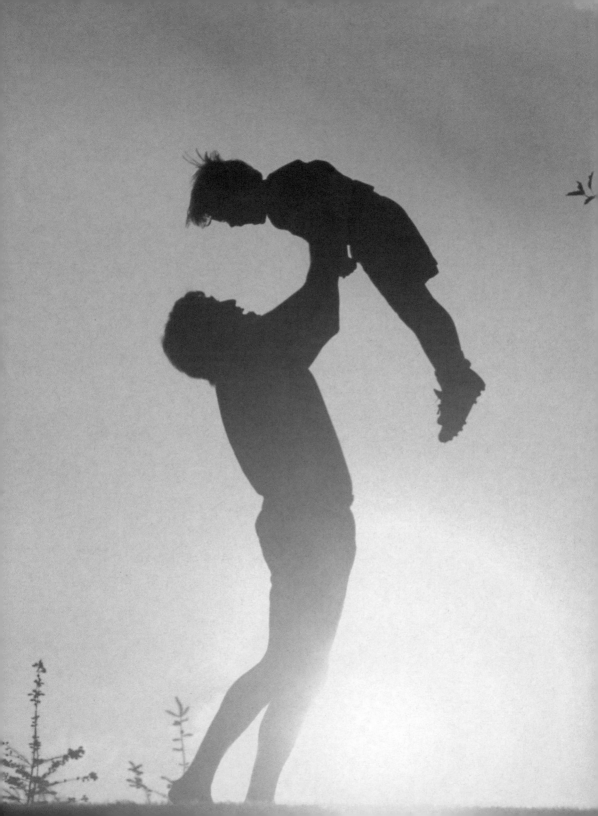

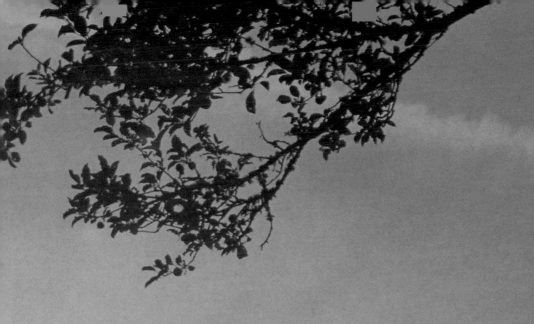

Support your body's natural ability to cleanse itself and eliminate the waste products of digestion and cell renewal, safely and easily.

Introduction ·

We live in an environment filled with toxins and pollutants. This causes contaminants to enter our body and become lodged throughout our tissues. The systems our bodies have evolved for detoxifying and passing poisons strain under accumulations of

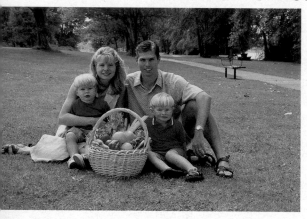

toxic waste. We are burdened with artificial colorings, pesticide and herbicide residues, preservatives, and rancid oils in our foods. We are unable to escape from dangerous, chemical-based cleaning products and cosmetics, out-gassing particleboards, harmful medications, and a host of other insidious poisons. Poor eating habits and lack of exercise have further clogged our system, thwarting our body's natural ability to cleanse itself and eliminate the waste products of digestion and cell renewal.

If the external toxins we acquire from our environment and the internal toxins we naturally produce can be eliminated in a timely manner, our health will be maintained. However, the over-accumulation of waste products and toxins in our cells, tissues, and organs interferes with the nourishment and oxygenation of these tissues, leaving the body weak and susceptible to disease. This chronic excess of toxins negatively impacts our health and robs us of vitality, clear thinking, and the robust life that is our potential. Therefore, it is important that environmental toxins and cell wastes are eliminated from the body as quickly and efficiently as possible.

Despite all the unavoidable contaminants we are exposed to, there is a way to take control of our health. Cleansing boosts our health by

- cleaning out the digestive tract
- clearing tissues of toxic substances
- increasing circulation
- eliminating toxin-producing foods
- creating a healthful life

Why Cleanse? . . . .

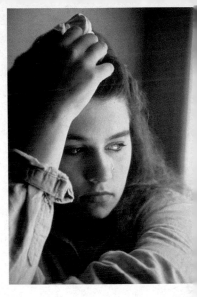

A mind-boggling number and variety of symptoms can be triggered by toxic overload. Accumulated bowel toxicity has led naturopathic doctors to trace more than 70 ailments to toxic bowels, including difficult-to-quantify symptoms, such as:

- Appendicitis
- Bad dreams
- High blood pressure
- Low blood pressure
- Bloating
- Constipation
- Drowsiness

- Fallen arches
- Fatigue
- Heart arrythmias
- Insomnia
- Unclean thoughts
- Tumors

Americans are exposed to an incredible amount of industrial pollutants, pesticides, herbicides, and synthetic chemicals. Today, nearly 900 active ingredients are found in our food, water, homes, schools, and workplaces. These are part of a larger chemical soup of over 60,000 commercially produced synthetic chemicals with about 1,000 new synthetic chemicals being released each year. These all build up in the body, and the cumulative effects have been shown to include:

- Cancer
- Immune system depression
- Contaminated breast milk
- Disruptions in the nervous system
- Reduced sperm counts, quality, and formation

There are two strategies we can take to manage the toxin onslaught:

1. Steer clear of environmental contaminants and avoid eating the dangerous chemicals found in and on food.

2. Change our internal chemistry to eliminate toxins already present in the body.

Implementing these strategies is as simple as cleaning up our diets by eating only whole organic fruits, vegetables, beans and grains, and by cleansing our bodies by the fasting principles in my weekend cleanse plan. But before we can understand the importance of an organic diet and regular internal cleansing, we need to understand how our bodies work.

The Digestive Tract

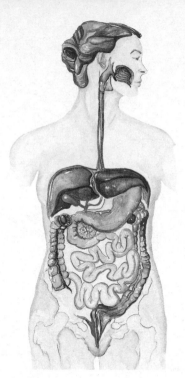

Food enters the mouth and is digested, absorbed, and eliminated—touching a universe of convoluted surfaces. Together, these surfaces form a large and primary interface with a vital source of life: the food we eat. During food's journey through the elaborate tube of our intestines, it is exposed to a cocktail of digestive enzymes. Each enzyme speeds up the reactions that break the food into usable molecules.

The role of digestion is to acquire materials and energy by digesting food into small molecules and then absorbing those molecules. Much of digestion is controlled by an autonomous nervous system—the "enteric" nervous system—that can function independently of the brain.

There are five processes that are involved with digestion:

- eating
- breaking down food into simpler chemical compounds,
- absorption
- assimilation
- elimination of waste

Our food choices play a significant role in the quality of our digestion. Although saliva and the process of chewing begin the process, the bulk of our food is broken down in the stomach and small intestine. Absorption is when molecules pass into our bloodstream. Assimilation is when those molecules enter our cells. Elimination of waste is the job of the colon, lymph, lungs, kidneys, and skin.

Start at the Top

For maximum digestion, food should be chewed thoroughly. Some macrobiotic sources recommend chewing each mouthful of food at least 50 times. That may be a difficult regimen to maintain, but even occasional counting of chews can be beneficial. Overstuffing the mouth and swallowing food before it is sufficiently broken down by teeth and saliva is a common source of mild indigestion and flatulence.

Saliva is rich in the enzyme called salivary amylase, which begins the digestion of starches. To get a sense of this, thoroughly chew a bite of bread, without swallowing, and taste the sweetness as the carbohydrates are broken down into sugars. Swallowing moves the chewed food down the esophagus, through a muscular door called the lower esophageal sphincter, and into the stomach.

Heartburn and Acid Reflux Disease

The continual bathing of the esophagus with stomach acid can cause chronic heartburn known as gastroesophageal reflux disease (GERD). Heartburn is often first felt as a burning sensation behind the breastbone that radiates up toward the neck. A sour or bitter taste may enter the mouth accompanied by a taste of the offending food. The discomfort from heartburn can interfere with sleep.

Overweight people are more likely to suffer from bloating, constipation, and gastroesophageal reflux disease than thin people. Excess weight increases pressure within and on the abdomen, forcing stomach acid up into the esophagus (acid reflux) causing heartburn and inflaming the delicate tissues lining the esophagus.

Noting which foods cause heartburn and avoiding them will reduce symptoms, as will quitting smoking and not drinking alcohol. Chronic acid reflux disease can lead to a number of worsening conditions such as Barrett's esophagus, erosive esophagitis, esophageal strictures, and esophageal cancer.

In the United States, heartburn has reached epidemic proportions, which has spawned a $13 billion-a-year antacid industry. But a study published in the Journal of the American Medical Association in 2004 casts doubt on the safety record of these drugs. The results showed that people who take antacids develop pneumonia four times more often than people who never took them. The reason appears to be that stomach acid protects the body from gastrointestinal pathogens, and the acid suppressants reduce the acid levels in the stomach. Just how pneumo-nia–causing bacteria and viruses move from the stomach into the lungs is not clear. The elderly tend to be the major consumers of acid-suppressing drugs, and for them, pneumonia can be deadly.

The Small Intestine

Digestive juices flow from the walls of the stomach, small intestines, pancreas, and gallbladder, releasing the enzymes, bile, and bacteria that break down our food. Enzymes break down complex molecules of fats, proteins, fiber, starches, and sugars (known as carbohydrates) into smaller, simpler strings of atoms. Deeper in the intestines, bacteria digest and release food nutrients. At some point, the size, structure, and content of the smaller nutrient molecules allow them entry into and through the 50 to 100 trillion cells that constitute the living wonder of our organs, nerves, and consciousness.

The activities of the stomach convert the food into a thick, soupy mass called chyme. Chyme releases most of its nutrients after leaving the stomach and entering the small intestine. The small intestine is a membrane moistened by mucus that protects the intestinal wall from digestive enzymes, provides a safe haven for the friendly bacteria, and lubricates the food, chyme, and feces passing through the digestive tract. The small intestine is also guarded by immune system cells to protect us from toxins that have passed through our mouths.

The surface of the small intestine is marked by 4 to 5 million small, finger-like projections called villi. These villi absorb the products of digestion (see the villus illustration on this page). Nutrients diffuse through the cells of the villi and pass through the capillary walls to enter the circulatory system and the lymphatic system.

There are three main sections of the small intestine: the duodenum, jejunum, and the ileum. The base of the stomach is gated by a sphincter muscle that relaxes and contracts, squirting small amounts of chyme into the first 12 to 18 inches of the small intestine that makes up the duodenum. Pancreatic juice and enzymes come in contact with

Intestinal Villi

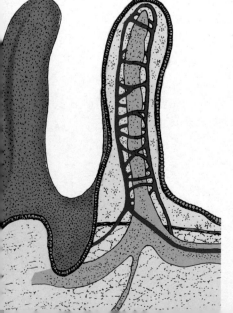

10

the chyme, releasing numerous nutrients into the blood.

The duodenum is where ulcers and other types of digestive stress can manifest. Sudden stress causes the adrenal glands to secrete hormones that reduce the supply of blood to the digestive tract and increase the blood supply to the muscles. Long-term, low-level stress can deplete the adrenal glands, wreck our digestion, and leave us with that "wiped out" feeling. Fortunately, stress-related problems usually can be reversed.

The duodenum is followed by 8 to 10 feet of thick-walled intestine known as the jejunum. Since most of the breakdown of foods happens before the beginning of the jejunum, its primary activity is absorption. The tissue of the jejunum is rippled with folds rich in blood vessels that harvest proteins, amino acids, sucrose, maltose, lactose, and water-soluble vitamins from the chyme.

From the jejunum, the chyme passes into the longest portion of the small intestine, the ileum. The ileum is a narrow, thinner-walled tube with fewer folds and blood vessels than the jejunum, and passes cholesterol, vitamin B12, and bile salts into the bloodstream.

The Helper System

The processing of food and the elimination of wastes and poisons involve every system of the body. Three organs of critical importance to the digestive tract are the liver, gallbladder, and pancreas, but lymph and bacteria also contribute greatly to the smooth running of the digestive tract.

Liver: The liver is absolutely essential in breaking down food molecules, reconstituting nutrients, processing vitamins and minerals, and neutralizing poisons. The liver is as critical to detoxification as lungs are to breathing.

You can locate your liver if you put your left hand over the lowest ribs on your front right side. Beneath your hand, concentrated in your liver, is 20 percent of your blood. Half your body's macrophages, critical agents of

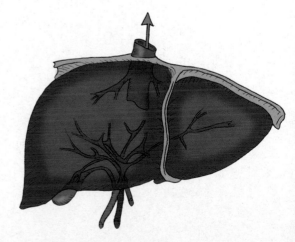

The Liver

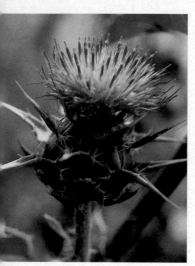

Natural compounds in milk thistle help support liver health.

your immune system, are located here. The liver maintains an astounding ability to regenerate itself—even if only 20 percent of it survives some calamity.

Both toxins and nutrients absorbed in the gastrointestinal tract are funneled into the liver. Toxic chemicals are met by 13,000 enzymes catalyzing hundreds of biochemical reactions that neutralize poisons. Research has shown that cruciferous vegetables and soy foods are rich in the enzymes necessary to help deactivate toxins in the liver. These foods include broccoli, Brussels sprouts, cabbage, cauliflower, kale, soymilk, tofu, and tempeh.

When these enzymes attach the toxin to a carrier molecule, that molecule is most often glutathione. The best sources of glutathione are raw vegetables and raw fruits. Foods richest in glutathione are asparagus, avocados, broccoli, garlic, okra, and spinach.

The powerful antioxidant milk thistle can prevent glutathione depletion. The active compound in this herb is silymarin, a natural liver detoxifier that protects the liver from poisons such as alcohol and carbon tetrachloride. Milk thistle is available as a supplement in most health food stores.

The liver, among its other functions, produces a green fluid called bile that breaks down molecules of cholesterol, fat, and fat-soluble vitamins into smaller globules so they can be more easily processed by the enzyme lipase. Bile flows from the liver into the duodenum. Additional bile secreted by the liver is stored in the gallbladder, which is later passed, as needed, through a narrow duct into the duodenum where it is quickly used for digestion. (See the illustration of the liver on page 11 and the pancreas on page 14.)

After nutrients have entered the bloodstream, they arrive at the liver. Some nutrients are stored there; others are assembled into more complex compounds, some of which form the liquid bile. Other nutrients and complex compounds are released by the liver and transported throughout the body, finding their way into the nourishing fluids that surround and bathe the cells. From there they enter the cell.

Sadly, 40,000 Americans die from liver disease each year. One of the best ways to keep your liver healthy is to not stress it. Some of the manufactured chemicals we ingest may be comparatively harmless, but others can be highly toxic. Although some chemicals are relatively easy for the liver to process, studies that examine the effects of the chemicals that find their way into our livers from processed food and industrial farming practices are difficult to conduct. To be safe, avoid synthetic chemicals in your food supply. Fried foods, such as french fries and fried chicken, are typically cooked in overheated hydrogenated fats. Foods like this place a heavy burden on the liver because they are sources of rancid fats and trans fatty acids. Rancid fats suppress the immune system and damage liver cell membranes. Trans fatty acids suppress production of the liver-protecting anti-inflammatory prostaglandin.

Alcohol is a challenging load for the liver and other parts of the digestive system. Alcohol inflames the lining of the stomach and can cause internal bleeding. Alcohol relaxes the lower esophageal sphincter, allowing stomach acids to flood the lower esophagus and induce heartburn. If a person is already suffering from diarrhea or nausea, even a moderate amount of alcohol will aggravate the symptoms. Heavy drinking over time is a leading cause of liver and pancreatic disease. Alcohol increases the possibilities of developing leaky gut syndrome, a condition where the mucous membrane is compromised and toxins and antigens enter the bloodstream. Abstention or moderation, even extreme moderation, is recommended, because anything beyond a moderate amount of alcohol is bad for the health. The Mayo Clinic offers these guidelines: "No more than one drink a day for women or two drinks a day for men. A drink is defined as twelve ounces of beer, five ounces of wine, or one and a half ounces of 80 proof distilled spirits."

Gallbladder: The gallbladder is a small, bag-like organ lying just below the liver, where bile produced by the liver is concentrated and stored. The gallbladder passes bile into the duodenum.

Bile is more concentrated and thicker in the gallbladder than it is when it flows fresh from the liver. This concentration is susceptible to the formation of gallstones, an especially painful condition. These crystal-like grains of cholesterol or calcium salts cause excruciating pain and vomiting when they become

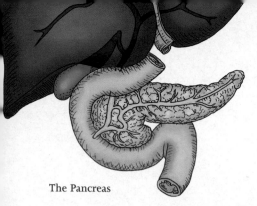

The Pancreas

lodged in the bile ducts entering the duodenum. While being overweight is a risk factor for gallstones, caution is urged when losing weight. Rapid or excessive weight loss can generate gallstone formation. Gradually losing weight at a rate of one to two pounds a week is less likely to instigate gallstone problems.

Pancreas: The pancreas is a six-inch-long organ resembling a stem thickly packed with ripe berries. The pancreas is primarily known for the production of the hormone insulin. The pancreas also produces enzyme-laden digestive juices that break down carbohydrates, proteins, and fats. These pancreatic enzymes are highly alkaline and neutralize the acidic chyme produced in the stomach.

Pancreatic enzymes enter the pancreatic duct that threads through the center of the pancreas and join with bile from the liver and gallbladder. If insulin regulation for blood sugar fails, people develop diabetes. Low secretion of pancreatic enzymes can lead to vitamin B_{12} nonabsorption and other nutritional deficiencies.

Colon: Chyme passes beyond the small intestine into the large intestine. Like the small intestine, the three to eight feet of the colon are considered in portions. (See the illustration of the large intestine on the facing page.) These are the ascending colon, running up the right side of the abdominal region; the transverse colon, traveling right to left from just beneath the lower forward points of the rib cage; and the descending colon, which follows. At the lower end of the descending colon is a horizontal twist called the sigmoid colon. The sigmoid colon is connected to the rectum and from there, stool leaves the body. The tissues of the large intestine are fed by powerful streams of blood beating from the heart into the aorta and through a series of arteries. The large intestine passes potassium, water, sodium chloride, and the products of colonic bacteria—vitamin K, short-chain fatty acids, and volatile fatty acids-into the blood.

A vast complex of blood vessels, lymph vessels,

After a good tweaking and purifying of the intestinal tract, the liver ought to be cleansed. The gentle way to do this is to eat liver-friendly foods that benefit liver function. Liver-friendly foods include a good number of whole grains, beans, fruits, and vegetables, such as: Beans, peas, lentils, seeds, brown rice, nuts, chocolate, whole grains, cold-pressed oils, avocados, garlic, onions, amaranth, kale, cruciferous vegetables, molasses, asparagus, spinach, leafy greens, citrus fruits, and juices.

14

and nerves surrounds the intestinal tract. A double layer of muscle wraps the intestine. The outer layer of muscle runs the length of the intestine, while the inner layer encircles the intestinal tube. In performing the work of mixing digestive juices and food moving the chyme along its path, the muscle layer gives form to the intestine. Inside the circular muscles are four layers of tissue: the submucosa, mucous membrane, the epithelium, and a coating of mucus called the lumen. Mucus smoothes the way for food and fecal matter to move through the system and supports friendly intestinal bacteria.

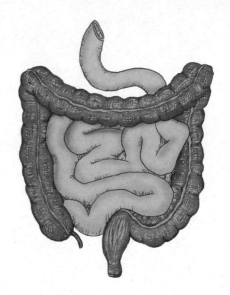

The Intestine

Intestinal Flora: Although not an organ, our gut microflora comprise an entire world within our intestines of trillions of microorganisms. They are as critical as the liver to cleansing health. The combined weight of the intestinal flora is about four pounds, just like the liver. Several ounces of new microbes are produced each day, while a similar amount is passed in the stool. Helpful bacteria are called probiotics; they guard against pathogens, synthesize vitamins, stimulate the immune system, and help to digest our food. (The term "probiotics" is also used to describe supplements containing helpful bacteria; these supplements are available in health food stores.)

More than 400 species of one-celled organisms live in our intestinal tract. Bacterial cells in our intestines outnumber all other cells in our body 10 to one. The bacterial density increases in concentration the farther down the intestinal tract we look. The importance of this internal ecosystem to our health cannot be underestimated. Not all of these bacterial cells are friendly or neutral. Some bacteria produce toxins, generate immune reactions, and can even aid the growth of cancer cells. The numbers of harmful bacteria are held in check by the abundance of friendly bacteria. Friendly bacteria also digest our foods and produce vitamin K and the B vitamins—folic acid, biotin, pantothenic acid, and B_{12}. We feed the bacteria and the bacteria feed us. The absurd idea of a "self" separate from the rest of life is exposed by our reliance on intestinal bacteria. Without this healthy collection of relationships, the individual dies.

The health of the intestinal microflora can be negatively affected by a variety of illnesses, dietary changes, and drug treatments—especially antibiotics. In some cases, where antibiotics destroy normal, health-promoting bacteria, there are life-threatening infections of dangerous bacteria. Beneficial bacteria, such as Lactobacillus acidophilus, grow in such tight colonies on the intestinal wall that pathogenic microbes, viruses, and fungi have nowhere to take hold. When antibiotics destroy Lactobacillus acidophilus, the body experiences an overgrowth of dangerous bacteria, allowing chronic, systemic disease to set in. A common example for women is the onset of vaginal yeast infections after taking antibiotics.

To make it through the upper digestive system and into the friendly parts of the lower intestine, probiotic supplements should be buffered with food and protected in the form of "prebiotics." Prebiotics are foods for friendly bacteria that pass undigested into the large intestine. Look for probiotic supplements with the prebiotics fructooligosaccharides (FOS) or inulin. Natural sources of FOS and inulin are asparagus, fruit, garlic, leeks, maple syrup, onions, soybeans, and, in smaller amounts, whole rye and whole wheat.

When the balance of the intestinal flora is disturbed by anything that reduces the amount of friendly bacteria, disease-producing organisms such as candida, clostridium, Hafnia alvei, and citrobacter flourish.

Lymph: The lymphatic system plays a major role in removing toxic proteins, absorbing fats from food, and fighting infections.

The powerful beating of the heart creates such an intense fluid pressure in the capillaries that water, proteins, and other materials leak out from the blood. This leaked nutrient-rich liquid is called the interstitial fluid. The cells of the body are bathed and nourished by the interstitial fluid, which seeps back into the capillaries with low fluid pressure. The rest finds its way back into the bloodstream by a route called the lymphatic system. When the interstitial fluid enters into the lymphatic system, it is called lymph. Lymph typically contains lymphocytes (a type of white blood cell that promotes immunity, called T cells and B cells), along with a wide range of waste from all parts of the body. Along the route lymph takes to and from the bloodstream are over 600 bean-shaped masses of tissue called lymph nodes, which filter out waste (especially bacteria) and prevent it from entering the bloodstream; the lymphocytes are allowed to pass through.

The heartbeat does not circulate the lymph. Lymph is moved by muscular contraction. Any vigorous aerobic exercise, massage, deep diaphragmatic breathing, and yogic postures—especially twisting—will help circulate lymph.

When the lymph system is overloaded with waste, the nodes can feel enlarged and tender. Tenderness indicates acute infection, while enlargement without tenderness indicates a chronic condition. Swollen lymph nodes can be indicators of serious diseases of the lymph system or even cancer. If you have persistent swollen lymph nodes, see a medical doctor.

Getting Things Moving . . . .

An efficiently operating large intestine is a foundation for health. Foremost, it passes waste from all other organs of digestion. Poisons, wastes, and most of the water that enters the digestive system are re-absorbed in the large intestine. Failure of the large intestine to re-absorb water results in diarrhea and dehydration. The intestine is vulnerable to great discomfort and disease (such as polyps and cancer) from the materials passing through it and from stress that originates elsewhere in the body. Fortunately, there are steps that can be taken to alleviate most intestinal health problems.

Constipation is the infrequent or difficult passage of hard, dry stools and is a source of extreme discomfort. The hardness of the stool, not the frequency of the bowel movement, is a primary indicator of constipation. One question that generates an incredible range of strong opinions is how often the bowels are to be moved. Once a day is the standard held by many Americans. Others call for a movement after every meal. A person may have two or three bowel movements a day or have one every

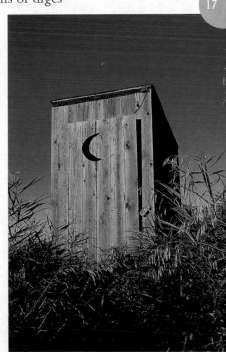

two or three days and still be in perfect health.

Stool should pass without discomfort or strain. Constipation slows bowel activity, allowing proteins to putrefy, fats to grow rancid, and sugars to ferment. When we are constipated, toxins that are passing through the system have longer periods of contact with the intestinal walls. Bile acids concentrate in the constipated bowel, irritating the colon wall. Hormones the body is trying to pass are re-absorbed and alter hormonal balance.

There are many causes of constipation; often they have to do with stress, activity level, and/or what, when, and how much we eat and drink. Certain medications or medical conditions can cause constipation. Temporary constipation is often related to emotional stress, travel, or a change in diet. Long-term constipation can be the result of poor bathroom habits, improper diet, difficulties scheduling toilet time during work hours or at crowded facilities, and so forth.

Mild constipation will usually pass on its own. For most people, the bowels will begin proper movement after a few days or a week. Try taking advantage of the first 15 minutes after breakfast, a time of high colonic activity, to move the bowels. The bowels usually move best following meals.

Stool Transit Time

If you like, you can perform an experiment to discover the transit time of your food Eat a cup or two of red beets. Note the time they are eaten. The beets will color the stool quite dark, often reddish to purple. Just watch for the color change in the stool to see how long it takes for the passage.

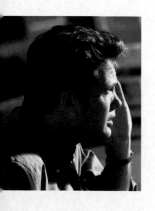

Medications

Most medications will have some effect on digestion. These effects can range from mild and unnoticeable, to constipation and internal bleeding. Many over-the-counter and prescription drugs create constipation as a side effect. Painkillers, such as those containing codeine and oxycodone, commonly cause constipation. Antispasmodics, antidepressants, and tranquilizers also contribute to the problem.

Some of the most commonly used over-the-counter drugs,

especially nonsteroidal anti-inflammatory drugs (NSAIDs), are among the most dangerous. This group of generally effective medications includes aspirin, ibuprofen, naproxen, and keto-profen, all sold under a variety of brand names. If they become a regular part of a person's self-treatment, or if used in excess of the recommended amount, they can cause stomach pain, ulcers, nausea, and diarrhea. Researchers at Baylor College of Medicine found an astounding 71 percent of patients who had been taking NSAIDs daily for three months for arthritis had ulcerations in their small intestines. Among 25 percent of the patients, the damage was deemed "severe."

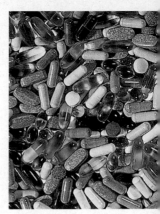

Other pain relievers, especially narcotics, can produce constipation. Blood pressure medications can cause diarrhea or constipation. Antibiotics can cause nausea or diarrhea while they are being taken. Additional problems can arise because the antibiotics destroy beneficial bacteria in the digestive system.

Disease

There are occasions when constipation is the result of common disorders, such as diverticulitis, or more seriously, cancer. Disease is likely the culprit if adults who have previously experienced regular bowel movements begin to have a persistent change in the character or frequency of their bowel movements.

There have been two studies linking constipation and breast cancer. A study reported in The Lancet involving 1,500 women showed that women having two bowel movements a week had four times the rate of breast cancer as women who had one or more daily bowel movements. Additionally, the researchers noted a few critical differences between the bowels of vegetarians and meat eaters. Meat eaters have greater amounts of cancer-causing substances in their bowels and, perhaps more specific to breast cancer, certain species of intestinal bacterial flora that interfere with the linkages needed to complete the excretion of estrogen introduced to the gut in bile. It is theorized that some of the "unlinked" estrogen is re-absorbed in the large intestine of meat eaters, possibly leading to higher estrogen levels and the subsequent growth of cancers with estrogen receptors.

Some naturopathic doctors assert that feces can harden and remain in the nooks and crannies of the large intestine for months and even years.

The mechanics of constipation cause their own sets of problems. The muscle strain used to pass difficult stools damages veins throughout the body-most especially creating hemorrhoids and varicose veins.

Change Your Mind

The first action you should take if you have constipation is to relax. Most instances of constipation will pass without worry or strain. It is important to create a relaxed and supportive toilet environment. Feng shui practitioners recommend the bathroom be kept clean and uncluttered. They encourage the "yang" of warm colors and the soft light of candles to promote balance and positive energy in this mostly "yin" environment.

A positive environment is conducive to clear thinking. The feedback mechanisms between the bowels and the highest potentials of the mind are so closely related that ayurvedic teacher Harish Johari considers care of the bowels to be preparation for spiritual practice. "Meditation can only be done when the stomach is clear and clean, when there are no toxins in the body. No meditation is possible if you have not been to the toilet." The late Swami Vishnudevananda agreed, saying, "Purity of the mind is not possible without purity of the body in which it functions, and by which it is affected."

When the urge to move the bowels is ignored, the sensation will pass. The addition of more food into the system will renew the urge. Consistent efforts to ignore the messages of the body will eventually cause the rectum to stop signalling. The resulting constipation can be severe.

Sometimes a large, hard stool can result in hemorrhoids or tear a tiny slit or fissure at the edge of the stretched anus. These tears can be quite painful. Bowel movements that follow can reopen the wound. Children who experience these can fear going to the toilet, generating more constipation and more painful movements. These painful conditions can cause even adults to further suppress the urge to defecate. A change in diet or a physician-recommended stool softener may be appropriate in these cases.

Some problems can arise when symptoms of a more serious ailment are diagnosed incorrectly. Pain is seldom associated with constipation. Assuming that abdominal pain is caused by constipation can lead to people dosing themselves with laxatives when the source of their pain may be something more severe, requiring immediate medical attention. Abdominal pain can also be caused by intestinal spasms that are perceived as abdominal cramps. Intestinal spasms often can be traced to emotional distress. Constipation may be associated with acute illnesses, old age, medications, or even simple cases of prolonged inactivity, poor food choices, or dehydration.

Be Wary of Laxatives

There are times when a mild laxative might be beneficial; however, there are real drawbacks. Consumer Union's The Medicine Show notes, "There can be no doubt that laxatives have contributed more to the ills and discomforts of mankind than the condition they are supposed to relieve." To purge the bowels when fluid reserves are already depleted can be disastrous. There are no perfect commercial products to alleviate constipation, and yet the laxative industry today boasts a cash flow of hundreds of million of dollars a year.

The body of any individual may react more or less strongly to a laxative. A laxative for one is a cathartic for another. The same person may react differently to the same dosage at different times. If you use a laxative, it is wise to use the least amount of the most gentle laxative that works.

When laxatives are employed to end constipation, a cycle of degenerating health may begin. Although the constipation that first inspires the use of laxatives can arise from myriad causes, continued use of laxatives brings changes in both the muscle tone and lining of the bowel. Extended use of laxatives can cause the natural muscular reflexes to diminish, requiring stronger doses of the laxative to move the bowels. Regular use of certain laxatives can deplete the body's supply of potassium, further weakening the muscles. After years of taking laxatives, the colon may be stretched into twisted coils that loop around to twice their original length. In those cases it may take days to fill the colon enough to stimulate a bowel movement.

Prunes, prune extract, and prune juice are wonderful ways to promote the contraction and relaxation of the intestines, propelling the contents along and ending constipation. Prunes are rich sources of fiber, vitamin A, and potassium. Potassium draws

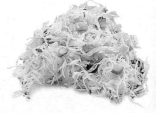

Sauerkraut is one of the many foods that can help relieve constipation naturally.

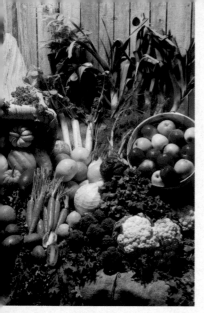

High-fiber foods help prevent constipation and provide many benefits for digestive health.

water into the fecal matter making it softer and easier to move.

The visionary physician John McDougall recommends, as a last resort for constipation, a nonabsorbable prescription sugar called lactulose. According to Dr. McDougall, lactulose draws water into the colon and helps to end constipation in even the toughest cases.

Fiber is critical in maintaining regular bowel movements. Including high-fiber foods as a regular part of the diet will go a long way toward warding off constipation. (See Nutrition Basics, page 27.) There are fiber supplements that should be taken with plenty of water. Some supplements are mostly bran; others contain methylcellulose or psyllium. Some people get temporary relief from constipation with magnesium–containing laxatives, but they can cause magnesium and sodium overload in older adults with renal dysfunction.

Hydrotherapy

Enemas can be effective for some people as an alternative to laxatives. A common and safe enema consists of a pint of tepid water introduced to the last eight inches of the colon. This can clean out old, hardened feces and get them moving. Enemas can create problems if used too frequently. Even once a week will be too much for some people. The problem, as with laxatives, is that the bowels will stop moving without periodic stimulation.

Enemas should be distinguished from colonic irrigation, also known as colon hydrotherapy, a procedure where the large intestine is pressure-infused with water or other liquids that are introduced through the rectum. Colonic irrigation attempts to reach far beyond the first few inches of the colon flushed by an ordinary enema. "High colonic" is a loose term for colon hydrotherapy, flushing the large intestine with 20 or more gallons of liquid administered by a pump or gravity-fed device. I do not recommend this method of bowel cleansing. Current mainstream medical understanding in the Western world is in general agreement: colonic irrigation for health improvement is not only useless but also dangerous. The hazards of colonic irrigation include the danger of excessive fluid absorption, perforation of the bowel, and fatal infection.

Diarrhea: The Opposite Problem

Diarrhea is a condition of loose, watery stools. A proper diagnosis from a trusted health care professional is essential if diarrhea lasts longer than one day or if there is fever, severe abdominal pains, or bloody stool. Although most viral attacks of diarrhea run their course in a couple days, some may last more than a week. There are many causes of diarrhea, including the use of antibiotics or other medications. Even doses of vitamin C can promote diarrhea. Diarrhea may be a symptom of more serious conditions, such as amoebic dysentery or ulcerative colitis.

Diarrhea can even occur when the bowel becomes impacted with feces. Impacted feces in the bowel is usually thought of as a form of constipation; however, with some conditions, such as irritable bowel syndrome, the body may liquefy the contents of the colon so that it passes through the compacted feces.

The treatment of diarrhea depends on its cause. A danger of diarrhea, regardless of its source, is dehydration. Fluid loss from diarrhea should be offset by drinking plenty of liquids. There are times when prescription drugs may be the best way to treat acute diarrhea.

Irritable Bowel Syndrome

Irritable bowel syndrome (IBS) is a disease that can affect nearly every part of the gastrointestinal tract. Irritable bowel syndrome is characterized by abnormal muscular contractions, especially a spastic colon, sometimes resulting in alternating constipation and bouts of diarrhea. The stool is likely to have excessive mucus. IBS is often associated with abdominal cramping, gas, bloating, and even a crampy urge to defecate without the bowels being moved. We do not know the causes of IBS and there is no certain cure. No sign of disease can be seen in the colon of a person suffering from irritable bowel syndrome, placing the disease in the category of functional disorders, where physiological functions are altered, rather than an identifiable structure or biochemical source being the problem. Although IBS is a serious cause of distress in and of itself, there is no evidence that it causes bleeding or permanent harm to the intestines.

The muscles that control contraction and relaxation (peristalsis) of the colon in people with irritable bowel syndrome seem to be extremely sensitive and reactive. This sensitivity causes the muscles to spasm in the presence of stimulation that would not bother most people. IBS symptoms can be triggered by gas, medications, particular foods, or even the simple act of eating. Eating normally stimulates the peristaltic action, but in irritable bowel syndrome the reaction is exaggerated. If medications and certain foods set the IBS symptoms in motion, they should be noted and avoided.

Emotions can trigger IBS symptoms, disrupting normal peristalsis and bringing on abdominal pain, distention, explosions of gas, and hard stools alternating with loose stools. The majority of people with irritable bowel syndrome who go to a gastrointestinal specialist are also dealing with some kind of emotional problem. Irritable bowel syndrome itself can be a significant source of emotional distress. When there appears to be an emotional component to IBS symptoms, it is important to at least cushion the anxiety and stress.

There are other causes of the symptoms normally found with IBS, so a diagnosis of IBS should not be assumed until the possibility of other conditions or diseases have been eliminated. For some, the cause may be food intolerance. Some people lack the intestinal enzyme lactase that is required to digest cow's milk and foods made from it. Other foods may cause episodes of similar discomfort.

There are ways to treat and manage the symptoms of irritable bowel syndrome. Relief can come from medications, dietary adjustments, and stress management. There may be times when lifestyle adjustments and dietary modifications will not be enough to control IBS symptoms. Your doctor or health care provider may recommend fiber supplements and/or medications to reduce cramps, spasms, and diarrhea.

Eat plenty of fiber, increasing the amounts gradually. Painful spasms may be reduced by the mild distention of the colon caused by fiber. Fiber can be supplemented by a gradual increase of fruits, vegetables, nuts, and whole grains. Brown rice is a nearly perfect food, as it is a whole grain high in fiber.

Eating too much food at one sitting can trigger IBS symptoms. Eat five or six smaller meals throughout the day instead of the more traditional three large meals. Eat smaller portions. Do not gobble food. Go slowly and try to avoid swallowing air. Drinking lots of water can reduce constipation.

Stress reduction can involve a wide variety of techniques, such as biofeedback, counseling, and exercise. Hatha yoga exercises and postures have been used for generations for relaxation, health, and spiritual awareness. There is mounting and compelling evidence that hypnotherapy is an effective treatment for irritable bowel syndrome.

Leaky Gut Syndrome

Leaky gut syndrome is the condition of increased permeability of the intestinal wall due to loss of the mucous membrane, or where the cells or spaces between the cells are compromised, permitting toxins and antigens to pass into the bloodstream. There are a number of causes of leaky gut syndrome, most of them having to do with the destruction of friendly bacteria and the overgrowth of disease-causing bacteria.

Problems with the intestinal wall and the bacteria enclosed within it play a complex role in the development of food sensitivity or intolerance. Food intolerance develops when the body reacts negatively to certain foods. It usually involves the digestive system and is marked by an adverse reaction when a particular food or ingredient is consumed.

Interspaced in the lining of the intestine are immune system cells. Some food proteins or disease-causing bacteria stimulate the immune cells to react defensively. This reaction is called an allergic response. The immune system treats the food item as an invasive toxin.

Alcohol consumption is a real danger. Even in amounts otherwise considered "moderate," alcohol can damage the intestinal membrane and encourage the overgrowth of harmful bacteria. Even healthy people have shown an increase in intestinal permeability after one shot of whisky. Worse yet, consuming alcohol and an allergen at the same time can intensify the allergic reaction.

There are other causes of leaky gut syndrome that are not clearly related to harmful bacteria. For example, chemotherapy used to destroy fast-growing cancer cells can increase the permeability of the intestinal wall. Treating cancers located on or near the intestines with radiation can also damage the intestinal wall.

25

Even moderate alcohol consumption can have detrimental effects on digestive health.

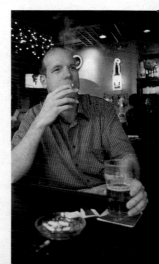

Colon Cancer

Colorectal cancer, commonly called simply "colon cancer," is the third most frequent cancer in the United States with approximately 150,000 new cases occurring annually, leading to about 57,000 deaths each year. Intestinal polyps are abnormal growths in the large intestine that can develop into colon cancer. Factors such as age, family history, obesity, diet, and lifestyle can all be significant risk factors for colon cancer.

There is growing evidence of a direct link between inflammation and colon cancers. The answer may be that inflammation and genetic mutation combine to turn healthy cells into malignant tumors.

When faced with an infection, large cells called macrophages mount part of the body's defense. Macrophages release cytokines—chemicals that induce more immune cells to flood the site of the infection. The immune cells not only destroy the pathogens, they also take out damaged tissue. One way the macrophages and other immune cells do this is by releasing highly reactive oxygen free radicals that can also destroy or damage DNA. If the DNA of a cell is destroyed, the cell dies. But if the DNA in a cell is only damaged, the cell may continue growing and dividing. This cell is abnormal but not necessarily cancerous.

Unfortunately, the immune system may treat the abnormal cell like a wound. Some cancer biologists assert that proteins and growth factors are brought in, flooding the abnormal cells with nutrients. This could cause the cells to develop into a tumor.

Some of these inflammatory cycles are well documented, such as the continual bathing of the esophagus with stomach acid, the condition known as chronic heartburn that predisposes people to esophageal cancer. Inflammation is one way the body removes toxins by killing off germs. Inflammation can also cause toxins to be diluted. The trick is to allow inflammation to do its work without causing damage.

Interestingly, studies have shown that patients who take anti-inflammatory drugs such as Celebrex and aspirin for conditions such as arthritis have less risk of developing colon polyps. These drugs are believed to block an enzyme that may trigger the development of polyps.

Our general health is intrinsically tied to the health of our digestive system, and the health of our digestive system is integrally tied to what we eat. Only the best food yields the best results.

Nutrition Basics . . . .

During our lifetime, each of us will consume an estimated two to three tons of food. The food we take in gives us the energy we need to carry on our daily activities. It also provides the nutrients we require to grow, repair tissues, and nourish our brain and all the systems of our body. It makes sense that we should eat the very best food we can.

Our bodies have the ability to balance caloric intake with caloric expenditure. But this balancing act can only work properly when the food going into our mouths is the food our bodies are adapted to process. In order to maximize our health, we must eat foods consistent with our digestive evolution: whole foods such as fresh fruits, vegetables, whole grains, beans, nuts, and seeds. Redesigning our menu in terms of the types of food we consume is more important than limiting portion size if we want to maintain this natural balance.

Some foods are critical to our health and pass easily and quickly through our system to help it function optimally. Plant foods are the ones to go for. Not only are whole plant foods rich in vitamins and minerals, they contain compounds that renew our bodies and protect us from cancer and other diseases. Fruits, vegetables, beans, and whole grains are also sources of fiber, which is vital to healthy digestion. These foods sustained our ancestors and were rich in both fiber and nutrients—mainly fruits, vegetables, whole grains, beans, and seeds.

Go Organic

A key to keeping dangerous toxins out of our bodies is to remove them from our surroundings. Most of these chemicals, an estimated 89 to 99 percent, gain access to our bodies through food. The foods highest on the food chain (meat, poul-

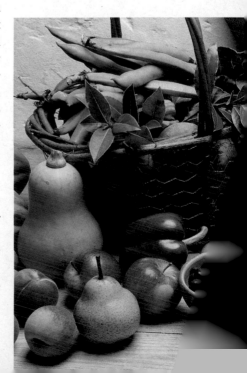

try, fish, and dairy products) are the foods with the highest levels of contamination. The reason is simple: The fatty tissues of these animal foods attract and concentrate chemicals. Toxins accumulate as they move up the food chain, resulting in a concentration of chemical threats.

Thoroughly washing and peeling plant foods can remove most surface contaminants. Unfortunately, many poisons used on agricultural crops are systemic; they work by entering into the cells of the plant. As there is no special labeling required, there is no easy way to tell if the foods we purchase in the grocery store have been treated with systemic poisons.

The clean-burning carbohydrates found in plants most effectively enhance the body's detoxifying processes. Meat, fish, poultry, and oil contain no carbohydrates. Undereating the right foods and overeating the wrong foods (and even eating too much of the "right" foods) almost invariably leads to a reduced capacity to deactivate toxic pollutants.

The most effective long-term change you can make is to eat organic produce that is untouched by herbicides, pesticides, fungicides, and petroleum-based fertilizers. Toxins concentrate in the tissues of animals, so avoiding fish and other animal foods will reduce your exposure to those chemical concentrations. Some toxins travel on cholesterol particles. Fortunately, there is no cholesterol in the plant kingdom, so a low-fat vegetarian diet can reduce the amount of cholesterol in the blood and minimize the toxins that are transported by it. Organic plant-based food is a critical component of cleansing.

What Is It About Fiber?

Humans process a variety of feedback mechanisms that signal when we have eaten enough food. One of the primary mechanisms to keep our digestion and weight in balance is the feeling of satiation—the sensation we feel as stretch receptor nerves embedded in the gastrointestinal tissues tell us how much the gut has expanded. Not enough stretch and we still feel hungry. Too much stretch and pain sets in. Another factor in this balancing act are nutrient receptors. Recent studies indicate that the human body has receptors for the three macronutrients—carbohydrates, fats, and protein—and these receptors trigger signals to the brain about the amount of nutrients that have been consumed.

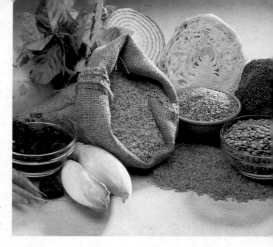

Fiber and water are essentially calorie-free. Carbohydrates and proteins are similar in caloric density; both contain about 1,800 calories per pound. Fat is the heavyweight in the macronutrient trio; it contains 4,000 calories per pound. In order to moderate our hunger drive, the body determines how much we have eaten based on our stomach's stretch sensation and the caloric density of the food consumed, and signals a sense of hunger or fullness. Additionally, the body monitors fat stores. When fat stores have reached adequate levels, the brain's appetite regulating centers are alerted, and the hunger drive is decreased.

Fiber is plentiful in traditional foods, such as beans and whole grains, as well as vegetables and fruits.

Our ancestral diet was probably 10 to 20 percent fat. Today the standard American diet is 20 to 40 percent fat. When compared to the standard American diet of 1980, Americans today eat 13 pounds more fat per year. While our diets were increasing in fat, why didn't our bodies signal the sensation of hunger to stop? How did Americans become so overweight? Lack of fiber is the culprit.

Carbohydrates provide us with two critical ingredients for healthy digestion—fuel and fiber. Cellulose, the most abundant molecule produced by living systems, is one type of dietary fiber. Cellulose fiber gives plant cells structural support. It is a major component of brown rice, whole wheat, carrots, leafy green vegetables, and most other plant material in our diet.

The current American diet has only a fraction of the fiber found in our ancestral diet. Although dietitians generally recommend getting 20 to 30 grams of fiber daily, most Americans get about 10 to 18 grams a day. Those who are eating a vegetarian diet are probably getting 30 to 40 grams of fiber per day. If vegetarians adhere to a dairy-free, egg-free vegan diet, the daily average is likely in the range of 40 to 50 grams of fiber.

Fiber is a major presence in the digestive system. By stimulating the stretch receptor sites in the gastrointestinal tract, fiber plays a role in how the body determines when enough food has been consumed. Prolonged consumption of foods low in fiber and high in fat disrupts this system; the result is an increase in

Avoiding Cancer

The results of several studies, reviews and meta-analyses support a significant reduction in the risks of colon and rectal cancers in association with the consumption of both fruits and vegetables. Additional studies show a relationship between increased fiber intake and lowered cancer risk, although the reasons are not clear. The role of fiber in producing anticarcinogens, diluting carcinogens, hastening the passage of carcinogens, and helping bacteria to limit the growth of cancer cells makes it an important weapon in the fight against cancer.

The same can not be said for meat, however: A review of 13 studies of the relationship between meat consumption and colorectal cancer was conducted by the University of Cambridge Institute of Public Health. The pooled results showed that as the amount of meat consumed daily increased, so did the risk for cancers of the colon and rectum. For processed meats, the picture is even bleaker: The risk grew by nearly 50 percent with a 25-gram daily increase in processed meats.

calories per volume of food ingested. With less plant fiber, there is less bulk relative to the number of calories consumed. Overeating is the immediate result. Continued overeating not only impairs digestion and bowel function, it also increases the risk of heart disease, stroke, diabetes, and obesity.

There are two forms of fiber: soluble and insoluble. Soluble fiber is most abundant in beans, oats, and fruit. Softer stools result from the consumption of soluble fiber because it absorbs up to 15 times its weight in water while moving through the digestive tract. Soluble fibers—such as mucilage, pectin, and gums—are partially broken down by our intestinal bacteria. These characteristics of soluble fiber are a gift to our digestive system, as the fiber helps sweep our intestines clean.

Stool receives its bulk from the insoluble fiber found in vegetables, legumes (peas, beans, and lentils), and whole grains. Plants are virtually our sole source of this critical dietary fiber. The only animal products with fiber are the membranes of some shellfish. As for red meat, chicken, eggs, and cheese, they contain no fiber at all. Refined flour and refined grains have had most of their precious fiber removed. People who adopt a vegetarian diet that includes whole grains automatically increase their intake of insoluble fiber.

The softening and bulking of stools produced by these two types of fiber help prevent a host of ailments, including constipation, some types of diarrhea, and some of the symptoms of irritable bowel syndrome. The passage of fiber actually reduces pressure on the intestinal walls, lessening the risk of diverticular disease and hemorrhoids. Cholesterol may be lowered as the liver creates more bile acids, which remove cholesterol from the bloodstream and cause them to be excreted into the stool. Diabetes may be better controlled with the consumption of fiber because fiber slows the release of sugar into the bloodstream. Although current research has not yet determined whether the benefit for those with diabetes is directly from the fiber itself or because a high-fiber diet is usually low in fat and high in nutrients that may help control blood sugar, the course of action is clear: Eat high-fiber foods.

When upping the fiber content of the diet, it is advisable to increase the amounts gradually. In certain circumstances, it is possible to have too much fiber in the diet. Too much too quickly can cause gas and bloating. Going more slowly will give the intestinal flora an opportunity to adjust.

In 1875 new milling techniques allowed the removal of bran and wheat germ from flour. The resulting white flour was a big hit with consumers who enjoyed the taste and texture. Manufacturers and grocery store owners liked the longer shelf life of processed grains and the concurrent increase in profitability. Unfortunately, the eliminated bran and wheat germ contained most of the fiber and substantial amounts of vitamins and minerals. In a short time, some of the negative health results of the new milling process became obvious, and iron and a portion of the B vitamins were added back into the flour. This attempt to replace the natural balance of nutrients in grains resulted in "enriched" flour, a product nutritionally inferior to whole-grain flour.

The Best Fluids

Drinking ample amounts of fluids is important for healthy digestion. Water is the best fluid, although most beverages, such as herbal tea and juice, are more than 90 percent water. The liquids that do not aid digestion are beer, wine, and hard liquor.

Fluids lubricate food as it passes along its digestive journey. Water-softened stools help prevent constipation. Fluids also increase nutrient absorption by dissolving minerals and fat-soluble vitamins such as vitamins A, D, E, and K.

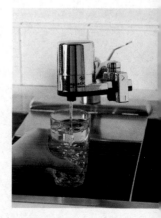

If you are uncertain if you are drinking enough liquids for good digestion, you can check the color and odor of your urine. A pale yellow color indicates enough liquid is going in. Dark yellow urine that smells of ammonia indicates a need to increase fluid intake. If urine is passed fewer than four times a day, more fluids are called for. If you have trouble urinating or if you are going so often that you are dehydrated, a health care professional should be consulted.

The Weekend Cleanse Plan . . . .

Many elements come together to support the cleansing process. We've covered some of the most crucial elements—pure nutritious food and regular elimination. These two factors alone will do wonders to help build a healthy body.

To round out the cleansing process, it's valuable to examine the mechanics of how to eat. This involves eating more slowly, chewing well, and appreciating your food. Breathing also comes into play, as the process of breathing cleans out toxins, and awareness of the breath settles the mind. Aerobics and resistance training will strengthen the body, encourage nutrients to do their work, and move toxins along their way.

One of the finest techniques for eliminating toxins is fasting. The weekend fast detailed in this book offers a method to begin using this valuable tool. You can skip a day or two of eating and come off a fast in better health than when you began.

All of these components—good nutrition, proper eating, conscious breathing, a supportive network, exercise, and fasting—are brought together in the Weekend Cleanse.

The Basics

The Weekend Cleanse is a simple two-day program of abstaining from solid foods and getting moderate exercise and plenty of rest. The Weekend Cleanse will release toxins, tune up the digestion, burn off a little weight, teach you important lessons about the body, and move you forward with improved health and digestion. The Weekend Cleanse is a powerful tool. It is not a cure-all, but it can rejuvenate the body and prevent the onset of illness. If the Weekend Cleanse becomes a turning point in how and what you eat, if it marks a new readiness to exercise, if the Weekend Cleanse gives you the confidence to make changes in your life and take personal control of your health, that is the measure of success.

Some of the beauty of the Weekend Cleanse is that it can be done without disrupting work schedules. Of course, certain weekend activities,

Exercise is one component of the Weekend Cleanse

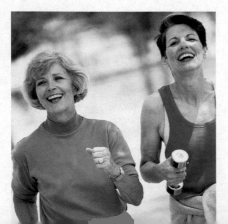

32

Cut the Fat

Excess fat in the diet slows digestion, causing heartburn, bloating, and constipation. Worse yet, excess fat raises our risk for a number of debilitating and even life-threatening health conditions such as heart disease, diabetes, and gallbladder disease. The symptoms of irritable bowel syndrome, pancreatitis, and Crohn's disease are all magnified by excess dietary fat. The exact mechanism is unclear, but research gathered by the American Institute for Cancer Research implicates dietary fat in the promotion of colon cancer, gallbladder cancer, and other cancers.

such as going out for dinner, may need to be postponed until a better time. Holidays, like Thanksgiving, when family and friends gather to eat in communion, are not good times for a cleanse.

The Weekend Cleanse should not be done by people with life-threatening diseases such as cancer, AIDS, hepatitis, kidney failure, or tuberculosis. Pregnant or lactating women, infants, and children should not do the Weekend Cleanse. Anyone taking prescription drugs should not undertake the Weekend Cleanse without first consulting with their doctor.

During the Weekend Cleanse, eat no fats, oils, starches, or meats. There are two drinking options for the weekend: water only, or liquids such as teas, Kicker Lemonade (page 44), and and/or fresh whole juices. Water is the simplest way to go. Our ancestors faced repeated and extensive periods of no food when only water was available. Our bodies have evolved complex and coordinated mechanisms of survival and healing in the absence of food.

The second decision is to choose when to begin and end the Weekend Cleanse. The best times to start are Friday evening after supper or Saturday morning after a light breakfast. Resume eating some solid food Sunday night or wait until Monday morning. I generally recommend waiting until Monday morning, but if you are new to fasting or have other reasons to eat Sunday night, go ahead and come off the fast.

The rest of this section explains pertinent details of the Weekend Cleanse. Take a look at The Weekend Cleanse: Day by Day (page 40), which shows where each of these elements comes into play.

Preparation

Plan to start your cleanse on a Saturday. Then you can begin preparing for the cleanse on Thursday or Friday. Sometimes there is a feeling of fatigue during the cleansing period. If that happens, limit activities that fall into the "must be done" category.

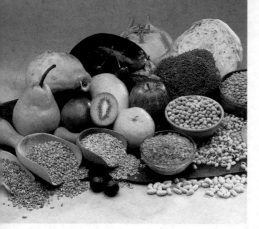

Be sure to have a supply of organic fruits and vegetables, along with brown rice, for coming off the Weekend Fast.

Try to rest without concern about accomplishing anything. Gather any foods or drinks you'll need for the next three days. If you're cleansing with water only, this will be easy. Also, have on hand foods for coming off the fast. This way they will be available should you decide to come off the fast sooner than planned. Purchase fresh organic fruits and vegetables. Make sure you have organic brown rice to prepare for coming off the fasting segment of the Weekend Cleanse. Portion out the drinks; plan on having juices and teas for Saturday and Sunday.

Friday afternoon and evening are good times to practice resistance training or aerobics. It's better to do a good workout on Friday and take it easy over the weekend. It's fine to do some gentle hatha yoga postures throughout the weekend of the cleanse. The increased flexibility you experience may be surprising.

Eat a light meal Friday night. Be careful not to overeat. Friday night is a traditional time to kick back and relax after a week of work, so relax your body. Relax your mind. Do not relax your awareness. Eat one helping of a balanced, well-cooked meal, seasoned to taste. Savor each mouthful. When finished, brush your teeth and scrape your tongue. Having clean teeth and tongue will help fend off the urge to eat after supper. Put away the food without picking at the leftovers. Wash the dishes. Clean the kitchen. Take a walk.

Fasting

Fasting is a well-established technique for removing toxins. When you fast, you purposely abstain from food for a limited time. Fasting has been proven to be effective for a variety of disorders of the stomach and intestines. Fasting improves the healing of diseases of the upper respiratory tract: the nostrils, nasal cavities, and sinuses. Fasting rests the digestive tract while activating stored toxins so they can be flushed from the body.

Fasting puts us in touch with our true sense of hunger. It is important to reconnect with the instinctual urge to eat because we have been socially and personally conditioned to eat types and quantities of food beyond what is needed for optimum health.

Fasting one day a week for a month or two can strengthen our understanding and physical ability to fast for the two fasting days of the Weekend Cleanse. Fasting is unwise and potentially dangerous for people with a compromised immune system, cancer, diabetes, gout, hypoglycemia, stomach ulcers, or disease of the liver, kidney, or lungs. People in these situations should only fast under direct medical supervision. Pregnant and lactating women should not fast, focusing instead on a healthful diet, exercise, relaxation, and loving relationships. Consult with a health care professional before fasting.

Fasting does not mean starving the body. Starvation is when the lack of food fuel causes the body to begin burning essential tissue in muscles and organs for energy. Extended fasts, in extreme situations, can lead to disturbances of the heart's rhythm and ultimately death.

During a fast, the body first utilizes carbohydrates stored in the cells as glycogen. As stored glycogen is depleted, the body begins harvesting fat as the preferred energy source. In this way, the protein in muscle tissue is partially spared. It is possible to lose some muscle tissue even during a short fast. The breakdown of muscle tissue will release ammonia and nitrogen into the blood. Additional stress can be placed on the kidneys by ketones, byproducts of fat metabolism, so it's important to drink plenty of water during a fast to help flush the kidneys.

The safest fast is short like the Weekend Cleanse, which lasts one or two days. Consult with a health care professional if there is any reason to think your health might preclude a fast. Even a healthy person wishing to fast more than two to three days should be medically supervised.

During a fast, persistent organic pollutants and other toxins that have been stored in the fatty tissues can be released. Concentrations of toxins passing into the urine and stool increase during a fast. The release of toxins can generate symptoms such as headaches, nausea, fatigue, weakness, depression, sweating, sore throat, runny nose, achy joints, palpitations, and dizziness. Although these may be side effects of fasting, they can also be caused by other serious medical problems. For this reason, it is important to have a health care professional you can consult while on a fast.

On one level, the presentation of symptoms is a good sign that the body is processing toxins. However, this is also a signal to slow down the cleanse. Drink some juice. If you still don't feel well after an hour or two, eat half a cup of cooked brown rice. If the symptoms pass, continue the fast. If the symptoms persist, gradually come off the fast by eating another half cup of brown rice or half a banana. Wait another hour or two and have more brown rice or banana.

Supplements and Medications

During the Weekend Cleanse, most common supplements can be skipped without ill effect. The best way to get vitamins and minerals is in their original package—fruits, vegetables, and whole grains. If you are concerned about missing vital minerals or vitamins, juice the vegetables or fruits that naturally contain those nutrients. People on medications should consult with their health care professional before trying the Weekend Cleanse.

Light Laxatives

My favorite laxative is psyllium seed husks. In our digestive tract, psyllium has attributes of both soluble and insoluble fiber. It is the most successful fiber for catching and passing toxins and cholesterol. Psyllium husks expand in water 10 to 15 times their weight to form a soft bulk that moves easily through the intestines. Mix one level tablespoon of psyllium husks in an 8- to 12-ounce glass of water to create a drink with a pleasant nutty flavor. Stir well and drink it before the husks settle. Continue to drink plenty of water until the bowels move.

Laxative teas are a soothing way to begin a cleanse. There are a number of laxative tea mixes on the market. I prefer teas made from only one herb so I can tell what that ingredient does to my body. Others may prefer a mix, either commercially available or a blend of their own choosing.

What to Drink

Tea: There are a number of pleasant, unsweetened teas you can sip during the two days of the Weekend Cleanse. In the evening, sip a cup of lemon balm tea, which is a calming seda- tive. Although the FDA recognizes lemon balm as safe, some herbalists suggest not operating motorized vehicles after drinking lemon balm tea. Not only is lemon balm itself a sedative, there is some evidence that it may increase the sedative effects of other drugs.

Milk thistle is a bitter tea that will rejuvenate the liver. It increases secretion and flow of bile with antioxidant properties and support for ribonucleic acid (RNA), working with DNA to bring about protein synthesis. The primary active ingredient in milk thistle seed is silymarin. Silymarin protects liver cells as they process toxins; it also helps to rebuild damaged liver tissue.

Peppermint tea is a pleasant, calming tea that will reduce nausea and settle the fasting stomach. Taken while not fasting, it aids in digestion and the reduction of flatulence.

Slippery elm bark makes a soothing tea that will reduce inflammation in the colon. Teas including slippery elm bark are available at most health food stores.

Coffee: Coffee can stimulate the bowels to move. If you are normally a coffee drinker, there is little harm in drinking a small amount of coffee in the morning. There are health promoters who argue vociferously against drinking coffee, as it can raise blood pressure and increase the risk of urinary tract cancer.

Whatever you decide about using coffee, carefully consider any reduction in consumption during your fast. For most heavy consumers of caffeine, the Weekend Cleanse may not be the best time to quit drinking coffee, although some may view this as an opportunity to shed a habit they have outgrown.

Water: For a steady fast, it is best to drink only water during the cleanse. Drink 8 to 10 glasses of water a day. Adequate hydration will help flush out disease-provoking toxins. The kidneys rarely pause in their efforts to wash fluid waste from the body, even during the Weekend Cleanse. On a normal day, the urinary system will filter 500 gallons of blood. The urine will pass environmental toxins converted by the liver and "cellular wastes" such as urea and ammonia produced during protein metabolism. The kidneys work hard and need water to function properly.

Juice: In modern times, juice fasting became popularized in Europe. A juice fast can easily transition a person into the fasting state of physiologic rest. Many people in relatively good health

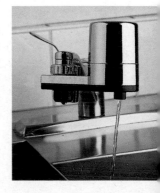

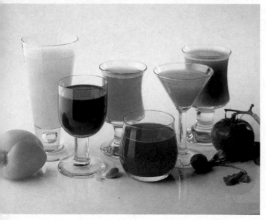

can stick with a juice fast for a longer period than a fast on water only. This is because juice provides an easily digestible and absorbable form of food for the cells of the body. Because of the ease of absorption, the digestive system gets a rest while the nutrient levels remain high.

Juice can be used for several purposes during the Weekend Cleanse. If you are fasting on water, you might want to switch to juice toward the end of the cleanse as a way to ease back into solid food, or you may feel you need the nutrients supplied by juice to carry on your activities during the Weekend Cleanse.

To accelerate the cleanse, drink a little organic fruit juice. Apple is a good choice. Organic cherry juice is my personal favorite for flushing out the system. It is nice to finish up on Sunday evening by drinking up to a quart of organic juice to clean out any intestinal residue that has accumulated over the weekend.

Freshly juiced apples are a rich source of the multipurpose health builder, fruit pectin. Fruit pectin cleanses the intestinal tract while lowering cholesterol and blood glucose. Although pectin is found in the highest concentrations in apples, it is also abundant in citrus fruits and is found to some extent in all fruits and vegetables. Beneficial intestinal flora thrives on pectin, helping to keep harmful bacteria and yeasts in check while synthesizing B vitamins. Pectin allows the helpful intestinal bacteria to produce short-chain fatty acids that act as a nutrient to the lining of the intestinal tract, protecting against cancer and upholding the integrity of the colon. Additionally, pectin helps the body to pass heavy metals such as beryllium, manganese, mercury, and especially lead.

Juice is the way to get concentrated nutrition in an easily assimilated form. Even if a person is suffering from weak digestion, juice will offer up 99 percent of the nutritional value of the produce it's made from. Try carrot juice. A pound of organic carrots will make a large glass of delicious carrot juice. We would have real trouble eating that many carrots but no trouble drinking all the enzymes, minerals, water-soluble vitamins, and trace elements extracted from that pound of carrots. During the week, juices provide the supplemental vitamins and minerals our bodies crave. During the Weekend Cleanse, they are essential foods.

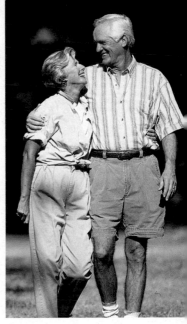

Listen to your body

Each day of the cleanse, take some time to be by yourself. Sitting with a straight, relaxed spine, close your eyes and observe your breath. See how your body is feeling. Pay close attention, especially during a cleansing process. A primary goal is to stay in touch with what your body is telling you. It is okay to stop a cleanse at any point and choose a new direction based on the feedback you receive from your body. If there are questions and the answers are not forthcoming, get the help of a trusted health care professional.

Get a good night's sleep. Sleep is critical to health. This is a time for the body to work at breaking down and eliminating wastes without serving the impulsive desires of the waking mind. If you experience fatigue during the days of the Weekend Cleanse, take a nap.

Coming Off the Weekend Cleanse · · · · · · · · · ·

By mid-week, you should be back to normal, eating the usual amounts of whole, organic, plant foods. But how food is eaten can be as important as what is eaten. Poor digestion can result from bad eating habits. Some of these habits may go on for years before the cumulative effects make themselves known. Digestion will improve if your awareness of what you eat and the feelings you experience as you eat translate into improved eating habits.

It is important to relax while eating. Eating in a hurry usually means inadequate chewing, swallowing more air, and experiencing heartburn, belching, bloating, and gas. Give food a good chew. Appreciate its taste. Avoid stressful situations while eating. Stress interferes with the normal activity of the intestines, causing a variety of "sick" stomach problems, including bloating and constipation or diarrhea.

Eat tasty food of high quality. But, as Grandma would admonish, "Don't let your eyes be bigger than your stomach."

Overeating is common everywhere in the world where people can afford to eat whatever they want, but the body is capable of producing only a limited volume of digestive fluids at any given time. Eating large amounts of food at one sitting puts a heavy burden on the digestive system.

The timing of food consumption is often regulated by the schedule of others rather the actual needs of our bodies. Eating on a regular schedule of our own choosing and regularly eating the same or similar foods aids digestion. An orderly entry ensures an orderly passage. People in the developed world who eat at regular intervals tend to eat more nutritious foods than those who eat at irregular intervals. Skipping meals can increase the appetite and lead to overeating.

The Weekend Cleanse: Day by Day

Friday evening

- Drink plenty of water
- Work out with weights
- Eat a light supper
- Brush teeth

- Long walk before bed
- Review goals and motivation
- Drink a laxative tea or drink
- Get a good night's sleep

Saturday morning

- Wake up and drink a glass of room temperature water
- Breathing exercises
- Shower
- Brush teeth

- Stretching and elimination exercises
- A little coffee, if that is the habit

Saturday (rest of the day)

- Drink plenty of water, juice, and/or Kicker Lemonade (page 44)
- Brush teeth
- Long walk before bed

- Shower
- Review goals and motivation
- Get a good night's sleep

Sunday morning

- Wake up and drink a glass of room temperature water
- Breathing exercises
- Shower
- Brush teeth

- Stretching and elimination exercises
- A little coffee
- Water, juice, and/or Kicker Lemonade (page 44)

Maintaining the Momentum . . . .

Some people like the effects of the Weekend Cleanse so much that they want to continue it for longer periods of time. Before experimenting further, however, please consult your health care professional.

In the meantime, you can maintain the positive effects of the Weekend Cleanse by eating organic plant foods, exercising, getting enough sleep, fasting one day per week, and cleansing regularly, up to five times a year.

Not all digestive problems can be prevented or controlled simply with lifestyle changes. Some conditions are hereditary; others are symptoms of infections or other causes, known or unknown. If your symptoms linger or become a daily annoyance, seek out the services of a health care professional. Often problems develop that would have been of little consequence if only they had been treated earlier. Sometimes problems can be avoided altogether just by following a sensible program of cleansing and renewal.

Sunday afternoon/evening

- If you have decided before-hand that you are coming off the fast tonight, eat a vegetable salad for supper.
- Long walk before bed

- Shower
- Brush teeth
- Review goals and motivation
- Get a good night's sleep

Monday

- Breathing exercises
- Drink a glass of room temperature water
- Light breakfast of brown rice or fruit salad
- Milk thistle tea or capsules
- Resume supplements about two hours after breakfast

- One or two cups cooked organic brown rice
- Stretching/elimination exercises
- Enjoy going to work
- Small lunch
- Small supper
- Walk before bed

Tuesday through Thursday

- Back to normal, if "normal" is eating a balanced plant-based diet with lots of fruit and vegetables. If not, now is the time to become a vegetarian.

- Eat sensibly
- Drink plenty of water
- Exercise
- Maintain positive outlook

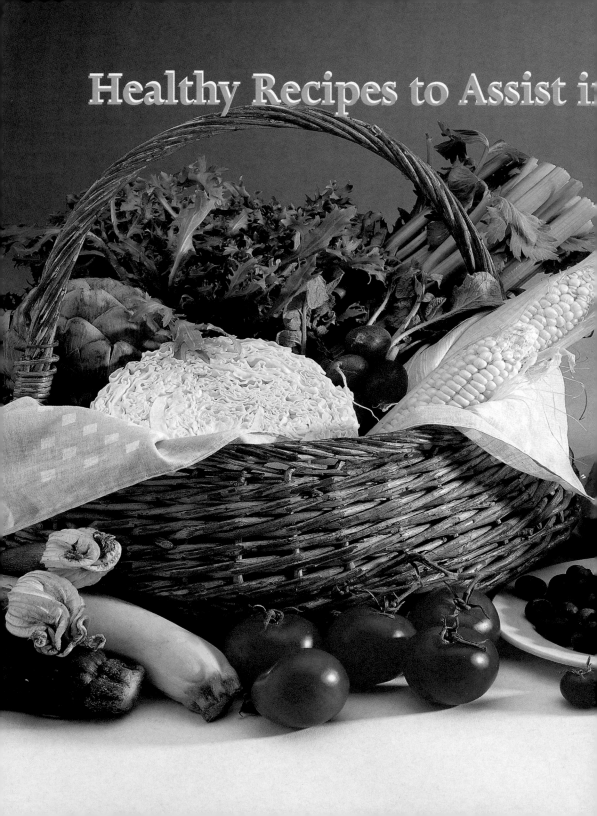

veryhighleansing

Juice provides an easily digestible and absorbable form of food for the cells of the body. Because of the ease of absorption, the digestive system gets a rest during a juice fast, while nutrient levels remain high.

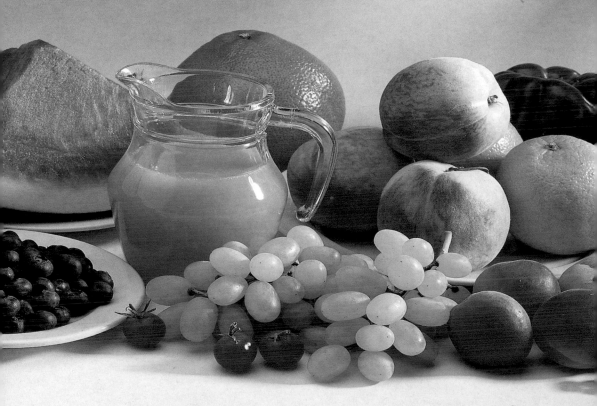

Kicker Lemonade

A glass of this invigorating drink will reveal how it gets the name! If you use honey to sweeten this, it will be absorbed quickly into the system and may be used in the Weekend Cleanse for short bursts of energy. People with diabetes should not use sugar or honey and should further consult with their heath care practitioners about all of the ingredients and methods used in a cleanse before beginning.

Juice of ½-1 large lemon

8 ounces water

1-3 tablespoons sweetener of choice (such as honey, maple syrup, agave syrup, sorghum syrup, or brown rice syrup-no sugar)

Pinch cayenne

There are a number of ways to prepare lemonade for a cleanse. Choose heavy lemons with thin skin and a bright yellow color; organic lemons are best. Wash the lemons thoroughly before cutting them open for juicing. Start with the juice of about half a lemon and adjust the strength to taste, adding as much lemon juice as seems appropriate. Do not drink so much that your belly hurts. Pain in the stomach area is an indication to back off the fast.

To spice the lemonade with a little "heat," add some mucus-dissolving cayenne.

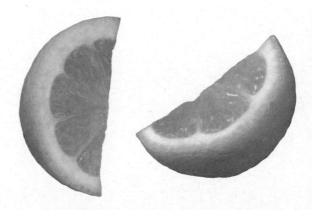

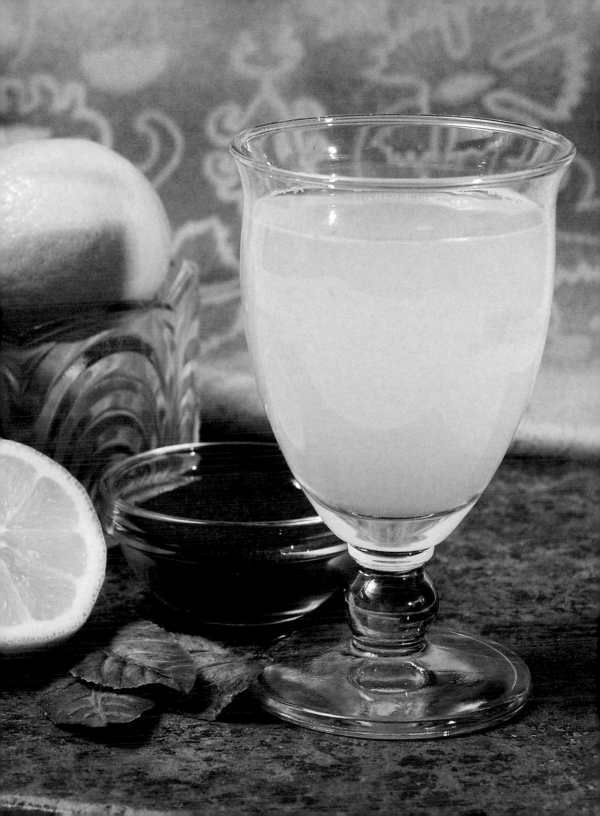

Fresh Quench

Using whole grapefruit segments when you juice will include the healthful fiber that is so good for digestion. Red and pink grapefruits contain more health-promoting antioxidants than yellow grapefruit.

5 oranges, juiced

1 grapefruit, juiced

2 lemons, juiced

½ cup ice (optional)

¼ cup pure maple syrup

Pour the juices into a blender. Add the optional ice and maple syrup. Blend for 4 minutes, or until the ice is pulverized.

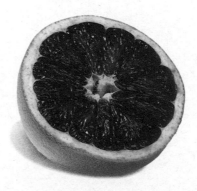

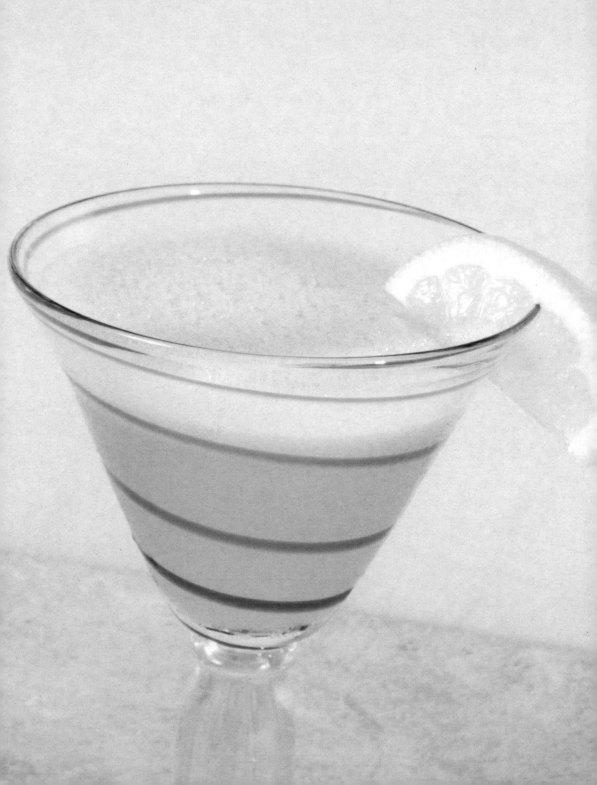

Apple-Sauerkraut Regulator

This is an effective remedy for constipation.

1 cup raw sauerkraut

4 carrots

1 Granny Smith apple

Process all the ingredients in a juicer.

Alternatively, combine in a blender with just enough water to enable the mixture to process easily. Strain out the pulp.

Variation:
Replace the carrots with ½ head butter or leaf lettuce.

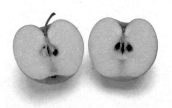

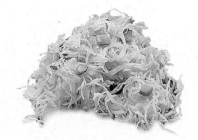

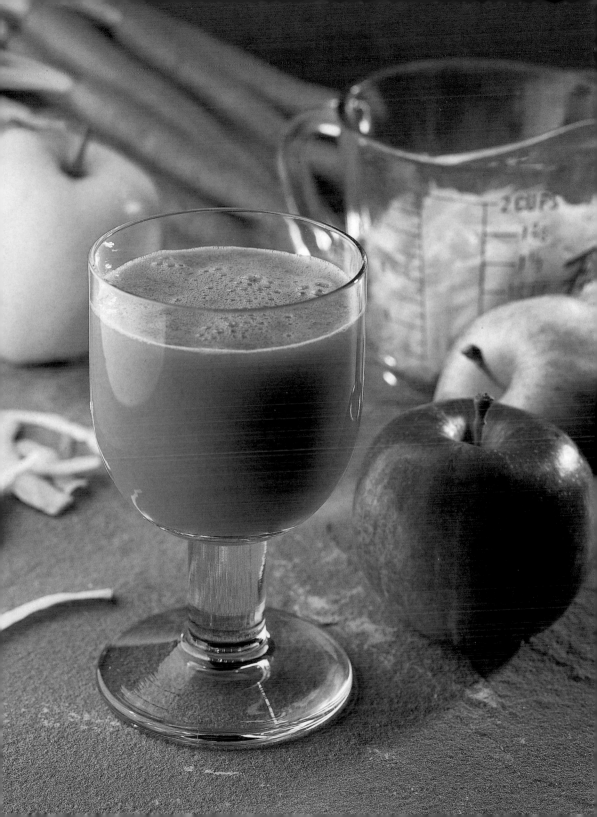

High Cs Smoothie

This combines fruits and vegetables with some of the highest vitamin C content.

I cup fresh orange juice

I cup fresh pineapple juice

I cup carrot juice

2 kiwis, peeled or unpeeled

I sweet red bell pepper, seeded and chopped

I teaspoon vitamin C powder (optional)

Blend all the ingredients until smooth. Serve immediately and enjoy.

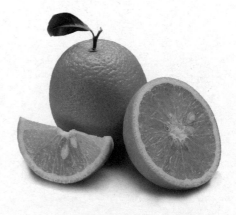

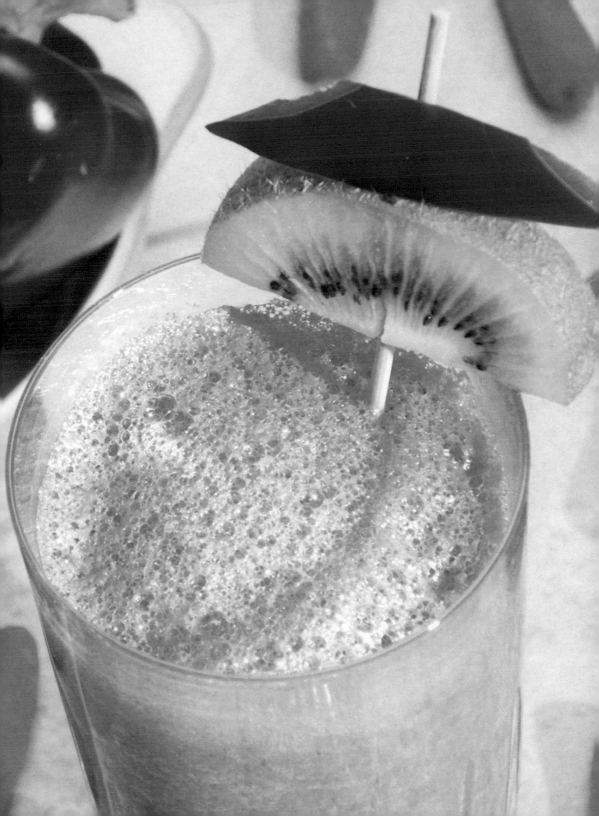

Black and Blue(Berry) Smoothie

Blueberries are a superfood, with a very high ability to reduce antioxidants.

1 cup frozen blackberries
1 cup frozen blueberries
1 cup apple juice
2 frozen bananas
1 tablespoon wheat germ

Blend all the ingredients until smooth and thick. Enjoy!

Variations
Substitute frozen raspberries or peaches for the blackberries.

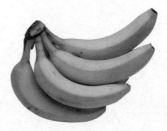

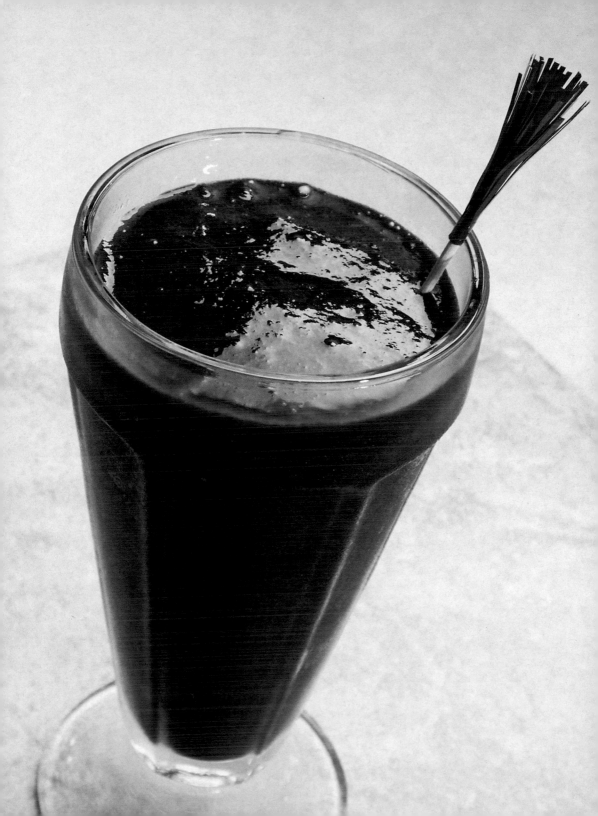

Carrot-Ginger Stomach Calmer

Ginger is well known in many traditional cuisines for its ability to cure indigestion and nausea.

2 carrots

1 stalk celery

1 raw potato

1 thumb size fresh ginger-root

¼ medium green cabbage

¼ fennel root

alternatively

1 medium papaya, seeded

3 slices pineapple

Process all the ingredients in a juicer.

Alternatively, combine in a blender with just enough water to enable the mixture to process easily. Strain out the pulp

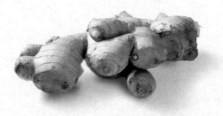

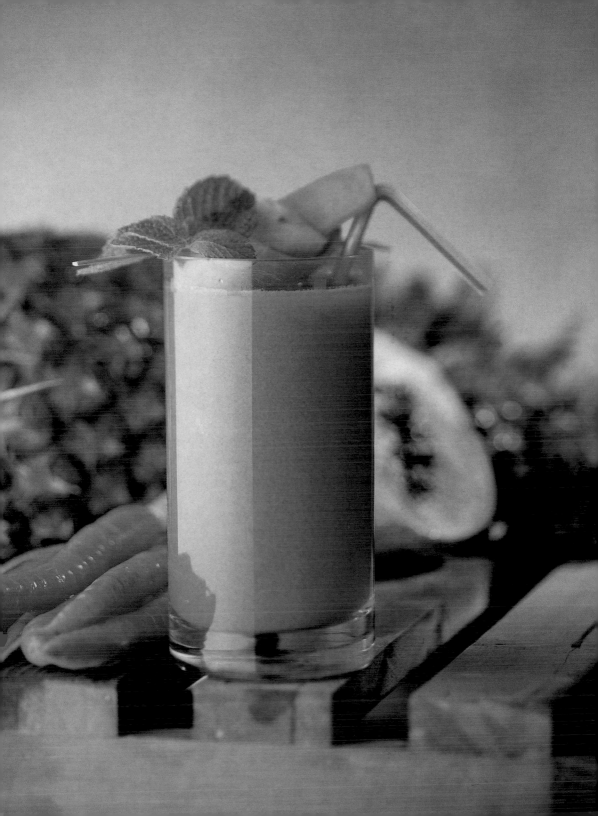

Vegetable Combo

One of the oldest and most versatile of the healing herbs, dandelion is regarded as a liver tonic, diuretic, and blood cleanser. Beets are one of nature's best bodily cleansers and detoxifiers.

2-3 carrots, juiced

1 cup spring water or distilled water

½-1 lemon, juiced

¼ beet, juiced

Pinch of dandelion (see note)

Combine all the ingredients in a blender and process until smooth.

Note: Dandelion is available in several forms: dried leaf, dried root, tea, extract (a powdered or liquid extract prepared from the roots, leaves, and flowers), and fresh leaves. A tea can be made from the dried root or from fresh leaves. For fresh tea, simply steam the fresh leaves like spinach and use the liquid they express as a tea. Any form of dandelion may be used in this recipe.

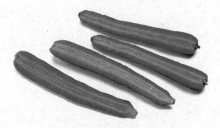

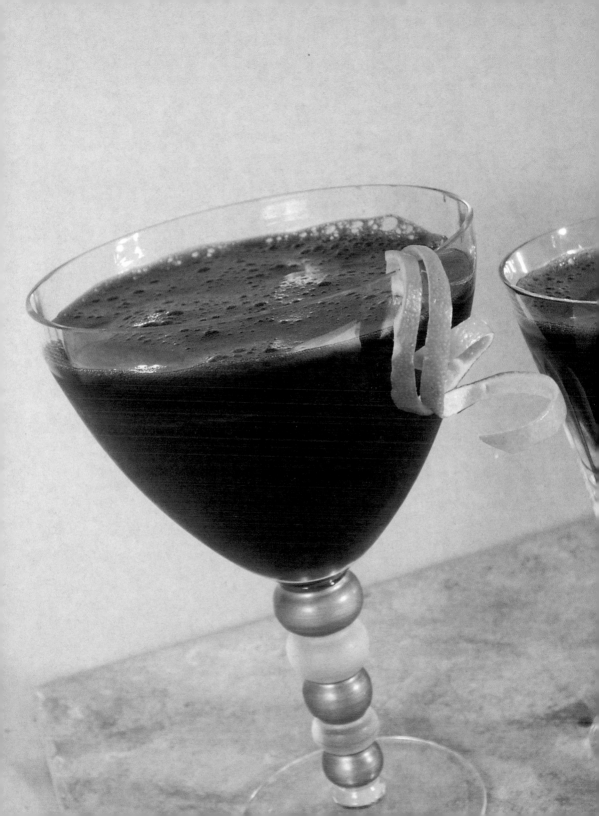

Asparagus-Radish Liver Tonic

Radishes, especially black radishes, help regenerate liver cells and stimulates production of bile. Asparagus contains large amounts of folacin which prevents liver disease.

1 black radish or 6-8 red radishes

12 large green and yellow leaves curly endive

6 stalks asparagus

3 carrots

1 cucumber

Process all the ingredients in a juicer.

Alternatively, combine in a blender with just enough water to enable the mixture to process easily. Strain out the pulp

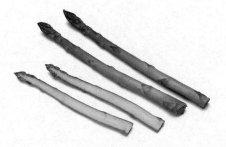

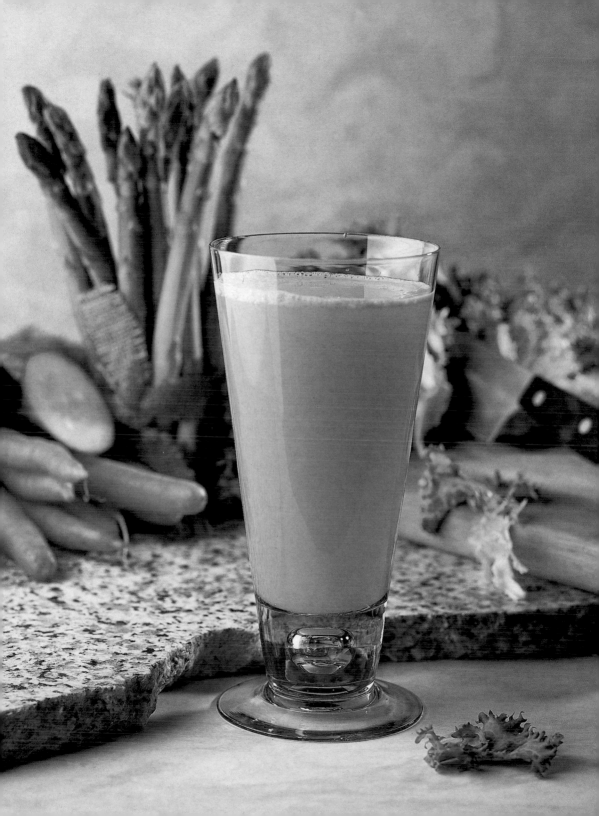

Celery Kidney Cleanse

Celery acts as a natural diaretic to help the kidneys cleanse excess liquid from the body.

3 celery stalks

2 tomatoes

1 lemon, peeled

2 carrots

6 large green leaves endive lettuce

Process all the ingredients in a juicer.

Alternatively, combine in a blender with just enough water to enable the mixture to process easily. Strain out the pulp

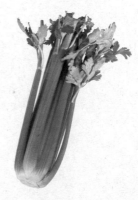

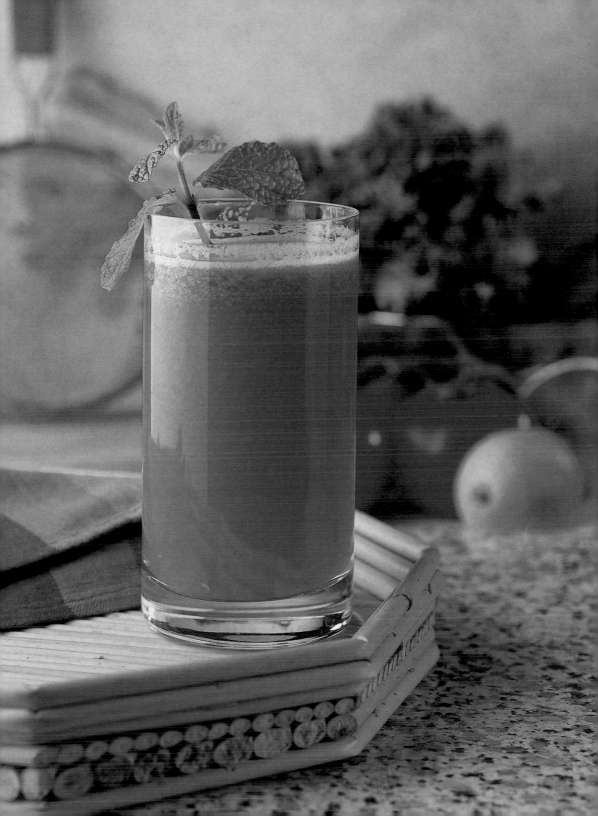

references

A.G. Andersen, T.K. Jensen, E. Carlsen, N. Jorgenson, A.M. Andersson, T. Krarup, N. Keiding, and N.E. Skakkebaek, "High frequency of sub-optimal semen quality in an unselected population of young men," *Human Reproduction* 15, no.2 (2002): 366-372.

Linda Berry, *Internal Cleansing* (New York: Three Rivers Press, 2000).

Cynthia Bye, "Reducing your toxic load," www.naturopathic.org/members/development/docs/reducing_toxic_loads.pdf

Brenda Davis and Vesanto Melina, *Becoming Vegan* (Summertown, TN: Book Publishing Company, 2000).

The Editors of *Consumer Reports*, *The Medicine Show*, (Mount Vernon, NY: Consumers Union, 1974).

E. Ernst, "Colonic irrigation and the theory of autointoxication: A triumph of ignorance over science," *Journal of Clinical Gastroenterology* 24, no. 4 (1997): 196-198.

W.M. Gonsalkorale and P.J. Whorwell, "Hypnotherapy in the treatment of irritable bowel syndrome," *European Journal of Gastroenterology and Hepatology* 17, no. 1 (2005): 15-20

R.J. Gilbert, "Pore-forming toxins," *Cellular and Molecular Life Sciences* 59, no. 5 (2002): 832-844.

Healing Edge Sciences, "The Amazing Liver: Liver Disease Risk Factors," www.healingedge.net/car_liver.html. Updated December 27, 2003.

K.A. Houpt, "Gastrointestical factors in hunger and satiety," *Neuroscience Biobehavorial Review* 6, no.2 (1982): 145-164.

Doug J. Lisle and Alan Goldhamer, *The Pleasure Trap*, (Summertown, TN: Book Publishing Company, 2003).

John McDougall, "A Cesspool of Pollutants: Now is the Time to Clean-up Your Body," *McDougall Newsletter*, 3, no. 8 (August 2004).

Vesanto Melina and Michael Klaper, "Creating and Maintaining a Healthy Intestinal Boundary," in Vesanto Melina, Jo Stepaniak, and Dina Aronson, *Food Allergy Survival Guide* (Summertown, TN: Healthy Living Publications, Book Publishing Company, 2004).

M.S. Micozzi, C.L. Carter, d. Albanes, P.R. Taylor, and L.M. Licitra (Armed Forces Institute of Pathology), "Bowel function and breast cancer in US women," *American Journal of Public Health* 79, no. 1 (1989): 73-75.

N.L. Petrakis and E.B. King, "Cytological abnormalities in nipple aspirates of breast fluid from women with severe constipation," *Lancet* 2, no. 8257 (1981): 1203-1204.

J.M. Samet, "What can we expect from epidemiologic studies of chemical mixtures?" *Toxicology* 105.

M.S. Sandhu, I.R. White, and K. McPherson, "Systematic review of the prospective cohort studies on meat consumption and colorectal cancer risk: A meta-analytical approach," *Cancer Epidemiology, Biomarkers, and Prevention* 10, no. 5 (2001): 439-446.

Weiss, B., S. Amler, and R. W. Amler. "Pesticides." *Pediatrics* 113, no. 4 (2004): S1030–S1036. See full text at www.pediatrics.org.

s o u r c e s

Juicers and equipment

Alpha Health Products Ltd.
7434 Fraser Park Drive
Burnaby, BC V5J 5B9,
Tel: 1-800-663-2212
www.alphahealth.ca

Tribest Corporation
1143 N. Patt Street
Anaheim, CA 92801
Tel: 1-888-254-7336, 714-879-7150
www.tribest.com

Published by **Books Alive**
PO Box 99
Summertown, TN 38483
(931) 964-3571
(888) 260-8458

Book Design:
  Paul Chau
Photographs & Food Styling:
  Warren Jefferson, Edmond Fong,
  Fred Edrissi
Artwork:
  Jerry Lee Hutchens
  Terence Yeung, Guy Andrews
Editing:
  Carole Lorente

Recipes courtesy of:

Juicing for the Health of It (Books Alive)
  Siegfried Gursche
Juice Power (Book Publishing Co.)
  Teoorah Shaleahk
Smoothie Power (Book Publishing Co.)
  Robert Oser

Library of Congress Cataloging-in-Publication Data
 Hutchens, Jerry Lee.
  Total cleansing : learn the secrets for effective detox / by Jerry Lee Hutchens.
    p. cm.
  Includes bibliographical references and index.
   ISBN 978-1-55312-044-5
  1. Detoxification (Health) I. Title.

RA784.5.H88 2008
613--dc22   2008015505

Printed in Hong Kong

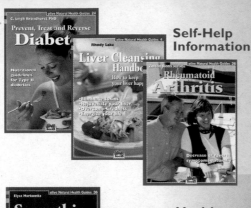
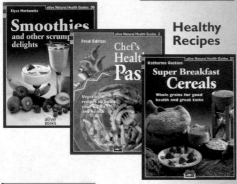
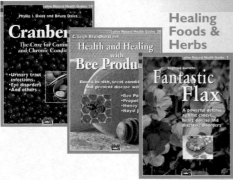
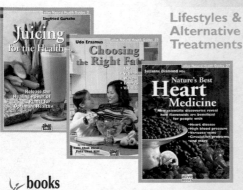
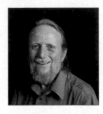